Contents

Eating and Diabetes

You can take good care of yourself and your diabetes
by learning

- what to eat

- how much to eat

- when to eat

Making wise food choices can help you

- feel good every day

- lose weight if you need to

- lower your risk for heart disease, stroke, and other
  problems caused by diabetes

Healthful eating helps keep your blood glucose, also
called blood sugar, in your target range. Physical activity
and, if needed, diabetes medicines also help. The
diabetes target range is the blood glucose level suggested
by diabetes experts for good health. You can help
prevent health problems by keeping your blood glucose
levels on target.

Blood Glucose Levels

What should my blood glucose levels be?

Target Blood Glucose Levels for People with Diabetes	
Before meals	70 to 130
1 to 2 hours after the start of a meal	less than 180

Talk with your health care provider about your blood glucose target levels and write them here:

My Target Blood Glucose Levels	
Before meals	_____ to _____
1 to 2 hours after the start of a meal	less than _____

Ask your doctor how often you should check your blood glucose on your own. Also ask your doctor for an A1C test at least twice a year. Your A1C number gives your average blood glucose for the past 3 months. The results from your blood glucose checks and your A1C test will tell you whether your diabetes care plan is working.

How can I keep my blood glucose levels on target?

You can keep your blood glucose levels on target by

- making wise food choices
- being physically active
- taking medicines if needed

For people taking certain diabetes medicines, following a schedule for meals, snacks, and physical activity is best. However, some diabetes medicines allow for more flexibility. You'll work with your health care team to create a diabetes plan that's best for you.

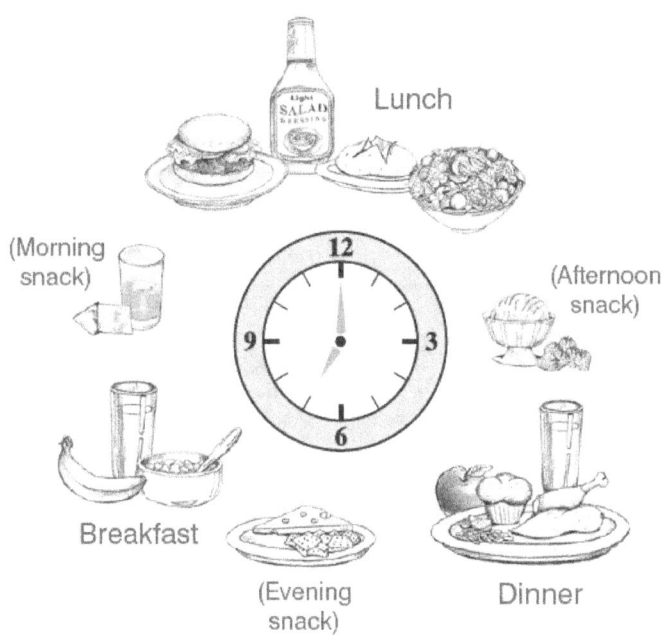

Talk with your doctor or diabetes teacher about how many meals and snacks to eat each day. Fill in the times for your meals and snacks on these clocks.

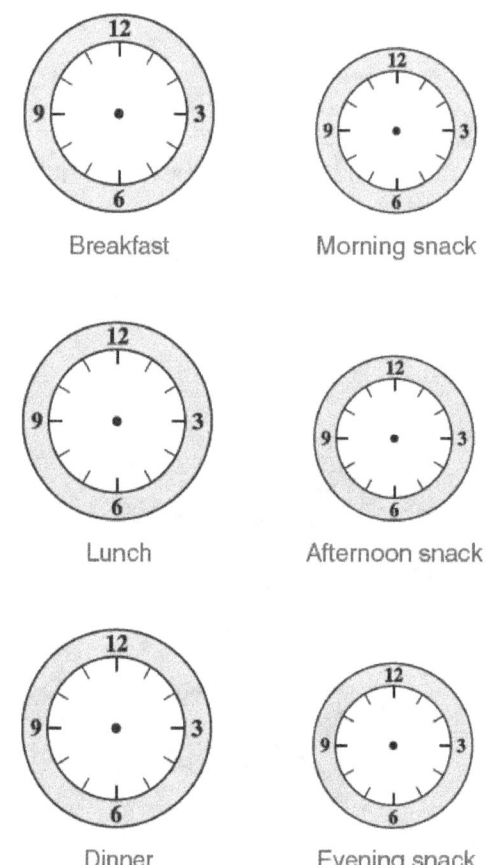

Breakfast

Morning snack

Lunch

Afternoon snack

Dinner

Evening snack

Your Diabetes Medicines

What you eat and when you eat affect how your diabetes medicines work. Talk with your doctor or diabetes teacher about when to take your diabetes medicines. Fill in the names of your diabetes medicines, when to take them, and how much to take. Draw hands on the clocks to show when to take your medicines.

Name of medicine: _____

Time:_____ Meal: _____

How much: _____

Name of medicine: _____

Time:_____ Meal: _____

How much: _____

Name of medicine: _____

Time:_____ Meal: _____

How much: _____

Name of medicine: _____

Time:_____ Meal: _____

How much: _____

5

Your Physical Activity Plan

What you eat and when also depend on how much you exercise. Physical activity is an important part of staying healthy and controlling your blood glucose. Keep these points in mind:

- Talk with your doctor about what types of exercise are safe for you.

- Make sure your shoes fit well and your socks stay clean and dry. Check your feet for redness or sores after exercising. Call your doctor if you have sores that do not heal.

- Warm up and stretch for 5 to 10 minutes before you exercise. Then cool down for several minutes after you exercise. For example, walk slowly at first, stretch, and then walk faster. Finish up by walking slowly again.

- Ask your doctor whether you should exercise if your blood glucose level is high.

- Ask your doctor whether you should have a snack before you exercise.

- Know the signs of low blood glucose, also called hypoglycemia. Always carry food or glucose tablets to treat low blood glucose.

- Always wear your medical identification or other ID.

- Find an exercise buddy. Many people find they are more likely to do something active if a friend joins them.

Low Blood Glucose (Hypoglycemia)

Low blood glucose can make you feel shaky, weak, confused, irritable, hungry, or tired. You may sweat a lot or get a headache. If you have these symptoms, check your blood glucose. If it is below 70, have **one** of the following right away:

- 3 or 4 glucose tablets

- 1 serving of glucose gel—the amount equal to 15 grams of carbohydrate

- 1/2 cup (4 ounces) of any fruit juice

- 1/2 cup (4 ounces) of a regular (**not diet**) soft drink

- 1 cup (8 ounces) of milk

- 5 or 6 pieces of hard candy

- 1 tablespoon of sugar or honey

After 15 minutes, check your blood glucose again. If it's still too low, have another serving. Repeat these steps until your blood glucose level is 70 or higher. If it will be an hour or more before your next meal, have a snack as well.

The Diabetes Food Pyramid

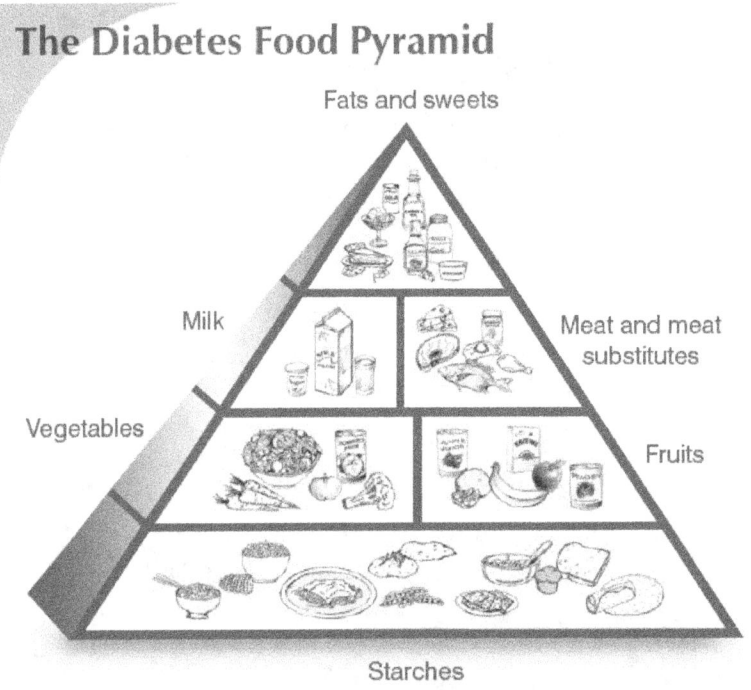

The diabetes food pyramid can help you make wise food choices. It divides foods into groups, based on what they contain. Eat more from the groups at the bottom of the pyramid, and less from the groups at the top. Foods from the starches, fruits, vegetables, and milk groups are highest in carbohydrate. They affect your blood glucose levels the most. See pages 9, 10, and 11 to find out how much to eat from each food group.

How much should I eat each day?

Have about **1,200 to 1,600 calories** a day if you are a

- small woman who exercises
- small or medium-sized woman who wants to lose weight
- medium-sized woman who does not exercise much

Choose this many servings from these food groups to have **1,200 to 1,600 calories** a day:

6 starches	2 milks
3 vegetables	4 to 6 ounces meat and meat substitutes
2 fruits	up to 3 fats

Talk with your diabetes teacher about how to make a meal plan that fits the way you usually eat, your daily routine, and your diabetes medicines. Then make your own plan.

Have about **1,600 to 2,000 calories** a day if you are a

- large woman who wants to lose weight
- small man at a healthy weight
- medium-sized man who does not exercise much
- medium-sized or large man who wants to lose weight

Choose this many servings from these food groups
to have **1,600 to 2,000 calories** a day:

8 starches	2 milks
4 vegetables	4 to 6 ounces meat and meat substitutes
3 fruits	up to 4 fats

Talk with your diabetes teacher about how to make a
meal plan that fits the way you usually eat, your daily
routine, and your diabetes medicines. Then make your
own plan.

Have about **2,000 to 2,400 calories** a day if you are a

- medium-sized or large man who exercises a lot or has a physically active job

- large man at a healthy weight

- medium-sized or large woman who exercises a lot or has a physically active job

Choose this many servings from these food groups to have **2,000 to 2,400 calories** a day:

10 starches	2 milks
4 vegetables	5 to 7 ounces meat and meat substitutes
4 fruits	up to 5 fats

Talk with your diabetes teacher about how to make a meal plan that fits the way you usually eat, your daily routine, and your diabetes medicines. Then make your own plan.

Make Your Own Diabetes Food Pyramid

Each day, I need

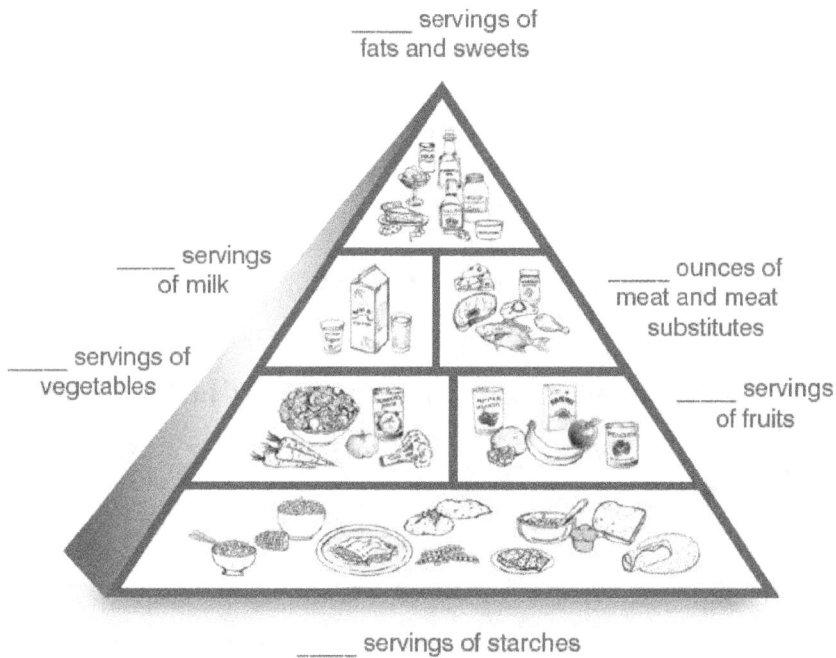

_____ servings of fats and sweets

_____ servings of milk

_____ ounces of meat and meat substitutes

_____ servings of vegetables

_____ servings of fruits

_____ servings of starches

On pages 38 and 39, you can make your own meal plan. Write down how many servings to have at your meals and snacks.

Starches

Starches are bread, grains, cereal, pasta, and starchy vegetables like corn and potatoes. They provide carbohydrate, vitamins, minerals, and fiber. Whole grain starches are healthier because they have more vitamins, minerals, and fiber.

Eat some starches at each meal. Eating starches is healthy for everyone, including people with diabetes.

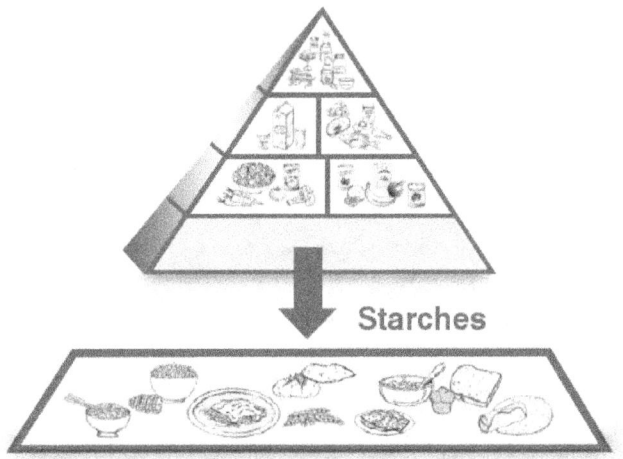

Examples of starches are

- bread
- pasta
- corn
- pretzels
- potatoes
- rice
- crackers
- cereal
- tortillas
- beans
- yams
- lentils

How much is a serving of starch?

Examples of 1 serving:

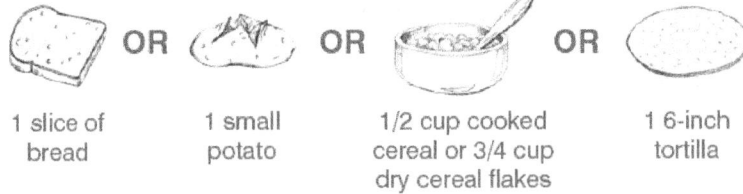

| 1 slice of bread | 1 small potato | 1/2 cup cooked cereal or 3/4 cup dry cereal flakes | 1 6-inch tortilla |

Examples of 2 servings:

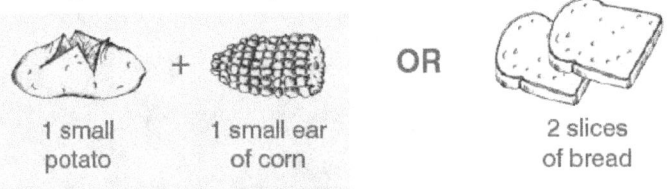

| 1 small potato + 1 small ear of corn | 2 slices of bread |

Examples of 3 servings:

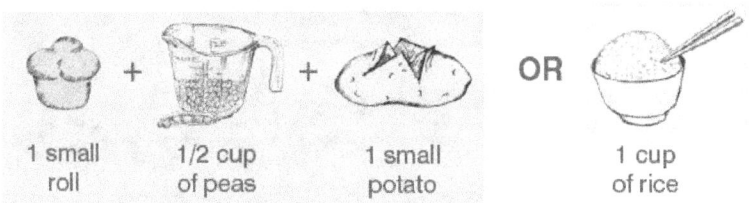

| 1 small roll + 1/2 cup of peas + 1 small potato | 1 cup of rice |

If your plan includes more than one serving at a meal, you can choose different starches or have several servings of one starch.

1. How many servings of grains, cereals, pasta, and starchy vegetables (starches) do you **now** eat each day?

   I eat _____ starch servings each day.

2. Go back to page 9, 10, or 11 to check how many servings of starches to have each day.

   I **will** eat _____ starch servings each day.

3. I will eat this many servings of starches at

   Breakfast _____   Snack _____

   Lunch _____   Snack _____

   Dinner _____   Snack _____

   A diabetes teacher can help you with your meal plan.

What are healthy ways to eat starches?

- Buy whole grain breads and cereals.

- Eat fewer fried and high-fat starches such as regular tortilla chips and potato chips, french fries, pastries, or biscuits. Try pretzels, fat-free popcorn, baked tortilla chips or potato chips, baked potatoes, or low-fat muffins.

- Use low-fat or fat-free plain yogurt or fat-free sour cream instead of regular sour cream on a baked potato.

- Use mustard instead of mayonnaise on a sandwich.

- Use low-fat or fat-free substitutes such as low-fat mayonnaise or light margarine on bread, rolls, or toast.

- Eat cereal with fat-free (skim) or low-fat (1%) milk.

Vegetables

Vegetables provide vitamins, minerals, and fiber. They are low in carbohydrate.

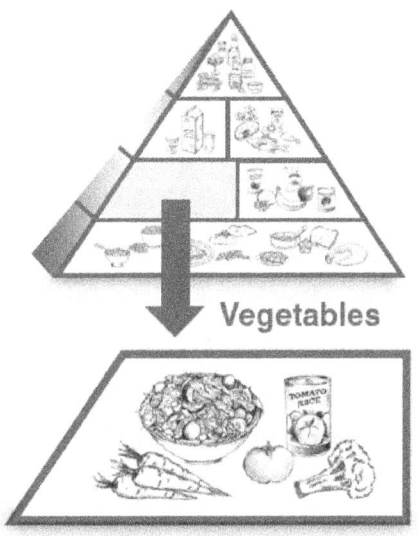

Examples of vegetables are

- lettuce
- broccoli
- vegetable juice
- spinach

- peppers
- carrots
- green beans
- tomatoes

- celery
- chilies
- greens
- cabbage

How much is a serving of vegetables?

Examples of 1 serving:

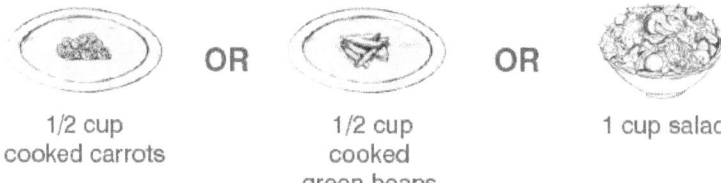

1/2 cup cooked carrots   OR   1/2 cup cooked green beans   OR   1 cup salad

Examples of 2 servings:

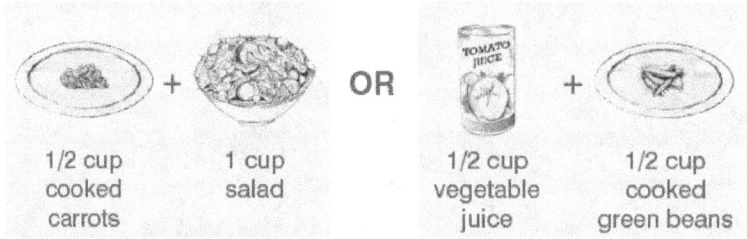

1/2 cup cooked carrots + 1 cup salad   OR   1/2 cup vegetable juice + 1/2 cup cooked green beans

Examples of 3 servings:

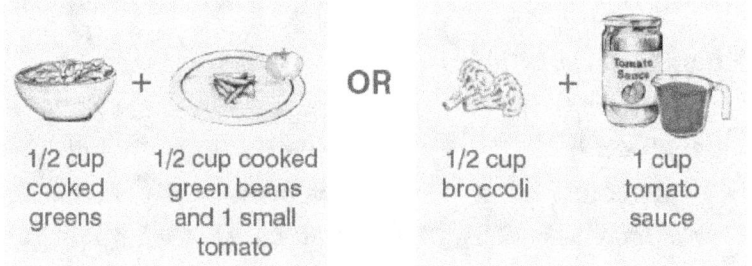

1/2 cup cooked greens + 1/2 cup cooked green beans and 1 small tomato   OR   1/2 cup broccoli + 1 cup tomato sauce

If your plan includes more than one serving at a meal, you can choose several types of vegetables or have two or three servings of one vegetable.

1. How many servings of vegetables do you **now** eat each day?

   I eat _____ vegetable servings each day.

2. Go back to page 9, 10, or 11 to check how many servings of vegetables to have each day.

   I **will** eat_____vegetable servings each day.

3. I will eat this many servings of vegetables at

   Breakfast _____   Snack _____

   Lunch _____   Snack _____

   Dinner _____   Snack _____

   A diabetes teacher can help you with your meal plan.

What are healthy ways to eat vegetables?

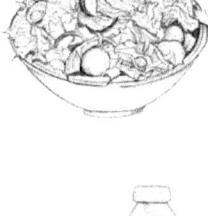

- Eat raw and cooked vegetables with little or no fat, sauces, or dressings.

- Try low-fat or fat-free salad dressing on raw vegetables or salads.

- Steam vegetables using water or low-fat broth.

- Mix in some chopped onion or garlic.

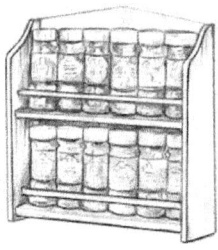

- Use a little vinegar or some lemon or lime juice.

- Add a small piece of lean ham or smoked turkey instead of fat to vegetables when cooking.

- Sprinkle with herbs and spices.

- If you do use a small amount of fat, use canola oil, olive oil, or soft margarines (liquid or tub types) instead of fat from meat, butter, or shortening.

Fruits

Fruits provide carbohydrate, vitamins, minerals, and fiber.

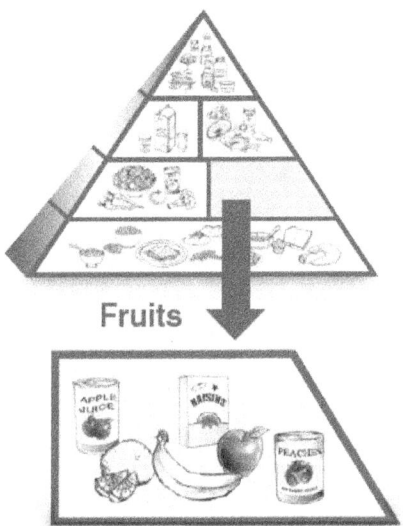

Fruits

Examples of fruits include

- apples
- fruit juice
- strawberries
- dried fruit
- grapefruit

- bananas
- raisins
- oranges
- watermelon
- peaches

- mango
- guava
- papaya
- berries
- canned fruit

How much is a serving of fruit?

Examples of 1 serving:

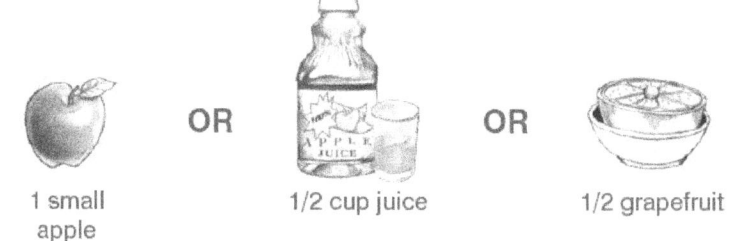

| 1 small apple | 1/2 cup juice | 1/2 grapefruit |

Examples of 2 servings:

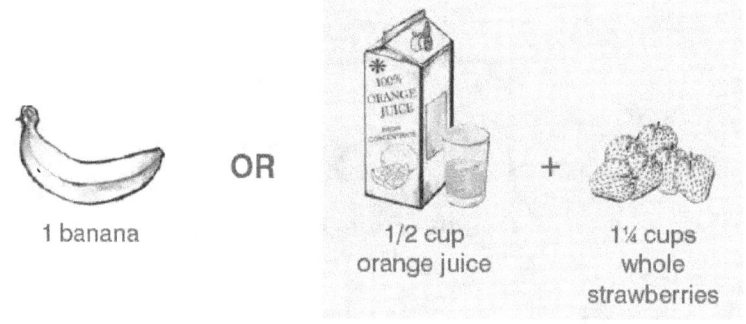

1 banana   OR   1/2 cup orange juice   +   1¼ cups whole strawberries

If your plan includes more than one serving at a meal, you can choose different types of fruit or have several servings of one fruit.

1. How many servings of fruit do you **now** eat each day?

    I eat _____ fruit servings each day.

2. Go back to page 9, 10, or 11 to check how many servings of fruit to have each day.

    I **will** eat _____ fruit servings each day.

3. I will eat this many servings of fruit at

    Breakfast _____   Snack _____

    Lunch _____   Snack _____

    Dinner _____   Snack _____

    A diabetes teacher can help you with your meal plan.

What are healthy ways to eat fruits?

- Eat fruits raw or cooked, as juice with no sugar added, canned in their own juice, or dried.

- Buy smaller pieces of fruit.

- Choose pieces of fruit more often than fruit juice. Whole fruit is more filling and has more fiber.

- Save high-sugar and high-fat fruit desserts such as peach cobbler or cherry pie for special occasions.

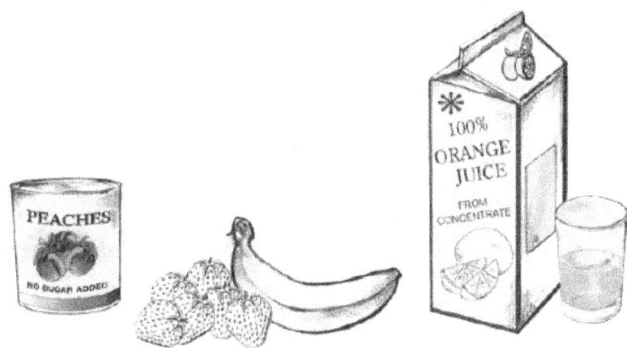

Milk

Milk provides carbohydrate, protein, calcium, vitamins, and minerals.

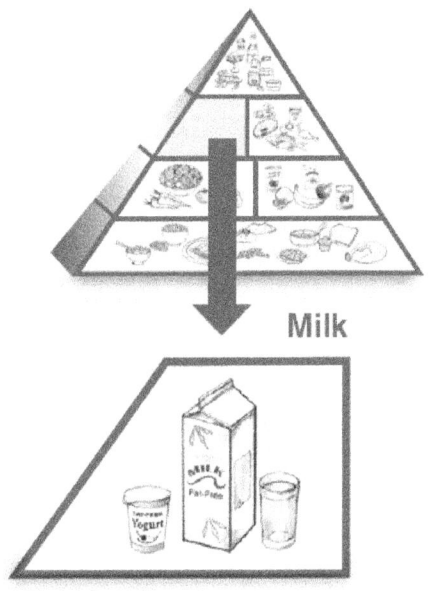

Milk

How much is a serving of milk?

Examples of 1 serving:

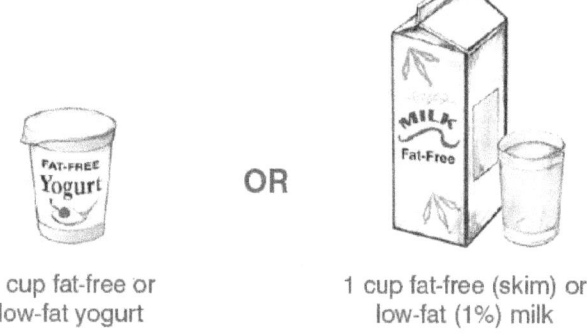

1 cup fat-free or
low-fat yogurt

OR

1 cup fat-free (skim) or
low-fat (1%) milk

Note: If you are pregnant or breastfeeding, have four to
five servings of milk each day.

1. How many servings of milk do you **now** have each day?

   I have _____ milk servings each day.

2. Go back to page 9, 10, or 11 to check how many servings of milk to have each day.

   I **will** have _____ milk servings each day.

3. I will have this many servings of milk at

   Breakfast _____   Snack _____

   Lunch _____   Snack _____

   Dinner _____   Snack _____

   A diabetes teacher can help you with your meal plan.

What are healthy ways to have milk?

- Drink fat-free (skim) or low-fat (1%) milk.

- Eat low-fat or fat-free fruit yogurt sweetened with a low-calorie sweetener.

- Use low-fat plain yogurt as a substitute for sour cream.

Meat and Meat Substitutes

The meat and meat substitutes group includes meat, poultry, eggs, cheese, fish, and tofu. Eat small amounts of some of these foods each day.

Meat and meat substitutes provide protein, vitamins, and minerals.

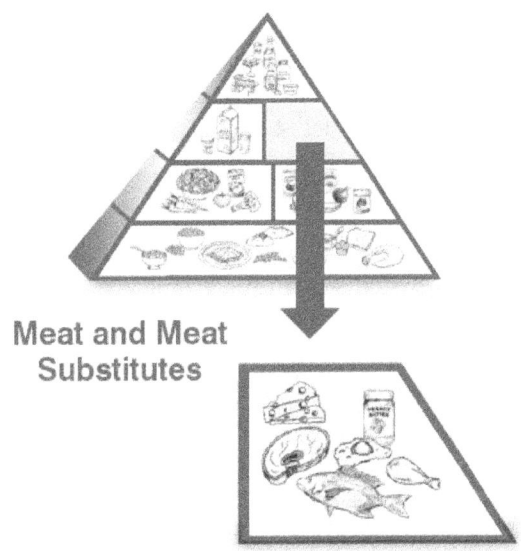

Meat and Meat Substitutes

Examples of meat and meat substitutes include

- chicken
- beef
- fish
- canned tuna or other fish

- eggs
- peanut butter
- tofu
- cottage cheese

- cheese
- pork
- lamb
- turkey

How much is a serving of meat and meat substitutes?

Meat and meat substitutes are measured in ounces. Here are examples.

Examples of a 1-ounce serving:

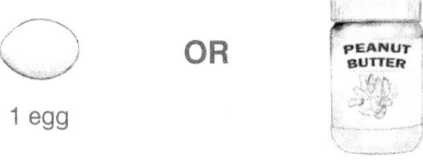

1 egg

2 tablespoons of peanut butter

Example of a 2-ounce serving:

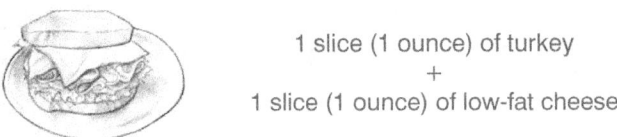

1 slice (1 ounce) of turkey
+
1 slice (1 ounce) of low-fat cheese

Example of a 3-ounce serving:

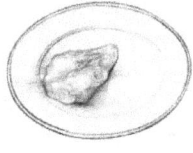

3 ounces of cooked lean meat, chicken, or fish*

*Three ounces of meat (after cooking) is about the size of a deck of cards.

1. How many ounces of meat and meat substitutes do you **now** eat each day?

   I eat _____ ounces of meat and meat substitutes each day.

2. Go back to page 9, 10, or 11 to check how many ounces of meat and meat substitutes to have each day.

   I **will** eat _____ ounces of meat and meat substitutes each day.

3. I will eat this many ounces of meat and meat substitutes at

   Breakfast _____   Snack _____

   Lunch _____   Snack _____

   Dinner _____   Snack _____

   A diabetes teacher can help you with your meal plan.

What are healthy ways to eat meat and meat substitutes?

- Buy cuts of beef, pork, ham, and lamb that have only a little fat on them. Trim off the extra fat.

- Eat chicken or turkey without the skin.

- Cook meat and meat substitutes in low-fat ways:
  - broil
  - grill
  - stir-fry
  - roast
  - steam
  - microwave

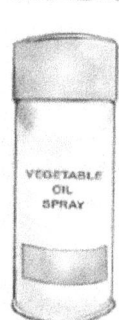

- To add more flavor, use vinegars, lemon juice, soy sauce, salsa, ketchup, barbecue sauce, herbs, and spices.

- Cook eggs using cooking spray or a non-stick pan.

- Limit the amount of nuts, peanut butter, and fried foods you eat. They are high in fat.

- Check food labels. Choose low-fat or fat-free cheese.

Fats and Sweets

Limit the amount of fats and sweets you eat. Fats and sweets are not as nutritious as other foods. Fats have a lot of calories. Sweets can be high in carbohydrate and fat. Some contain saturated fats, trans fats, and cholesterol that increase your risk of heart disease. Limiting these foods will help you lose weight and keep your blood glucose and blood fats under control.

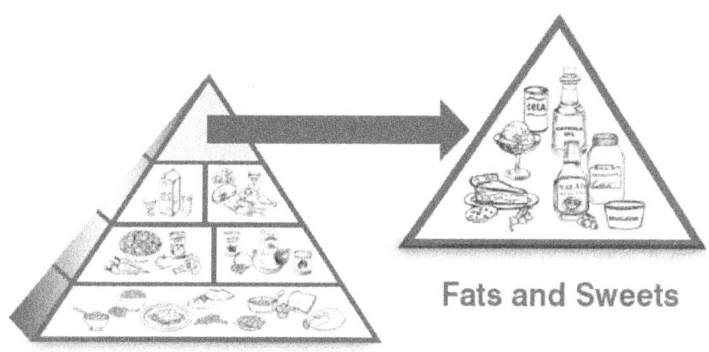

Fats and Sweets

Examples of fats include
- salad dressing
- oil
- cream cheese
- butter
- margarine
- mayonnaise
- avocado
- olives
- bacon

Examples of sweets include
- cake
- ice cream
- pie
- syrup
- cookies
- doughnuts

How much is a serving of sweets?

Examples of 1 serving:

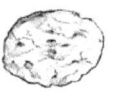 OR 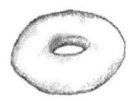 OR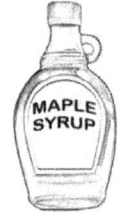

1 3-inch
cookie

1 plain cake
doughnut

1 tablespoon
maple syrup

How much is a serving of fat?

Examples of 1 serving:

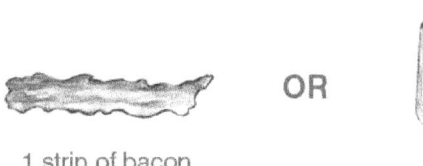

1 strip of bacon   OR   1 teaspoon oil

Examples of 2 servings:

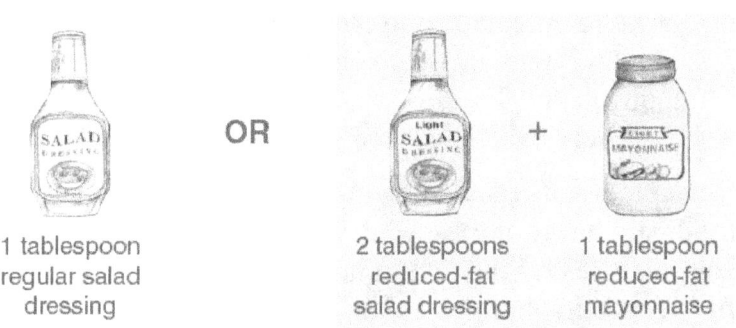

1 tablespoon
regular salad
dressing

OR

2 tablespoons
reduced-fat
salad dressing

+

1 tablespoon
reduced-fat
mayonnaise

How can I satisfy my sweet tooth?

Try having sugar-free popsicles, diet soda, fat-free ice cream or frozen yogurt, or sugar-free hot cocoa mix.

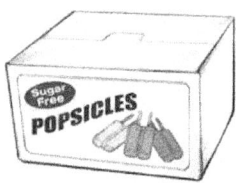

Other tips:

- Share desserts in restaurants.

- Order small or child-size servings of ice cream or frozen yogurt.

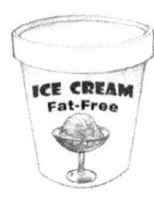

- Divide homemade desserts into small servings and wrap each individually. Freeze extra servings.

Remember, fat-free and low-sugar foods still have calories. Talk with your diabetes teacher about how to fit sweets into your meal plan.

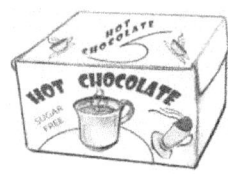

Alcoholic Drinks

Alcoholic drinks have calories but no nutrients. If you have alcoholic drinks on an empty stomach, they can make your blood glucose level go too low. Alcoholic drinks also can raise your blood fats. If you want to have alcoholic drinks, talk with your doctor or diabetes teacher about how much to have.

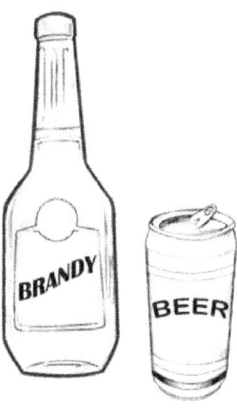

Your Meal Plan

Plan your meals and snacks for one day. Work with your diabetes teacher if you need help.

Breakfast

Food Group	Food	How Much

Snack

Food Group	Food	How Much

Lunch

Food Group	Food	How Much

Snack

Food Group	Food	How Much
_____	_____	_____
_____	_____	_____
_____	_____	_____

Dinner

Food Group	Food	How Much
_____	_____	_____
_____	_____	_____
_____	_____	_____
_____	_____	_____
_____	_____	_____
_____	_____	_____
_____	_____	_____
_____	_____	_____
_____	_____	_____

Snack

Food Group	Food	How Much
_____	_____	_____
_____	_____	_____
_____	_____	_____

Measuring Your Food

To make sure your food servings are the right size, you can use

- measuring cups
- measuring spoons
- a food scale

Or you can use the guide below. Also, the Nutrition Facts label on food packages tells you how much of that food is in one serving.

Guide to Sensible Serving Sizes

This much	is the same as

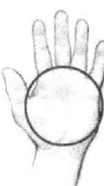

3 ounces
1 serving of meat, chicken, turkey, or fish

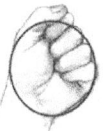

1 cup
1 serving of
- cooked vegetables
- salads
- casseroles or stews, such as chili with beans
- milk

This much	is the same as

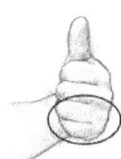

1/2 cup
1 serving of
- fruit or fruit juice
- starchy vegetables, such as potatoes or corn
- pinto beans and other dried beans
- rice or noodles
- cereal

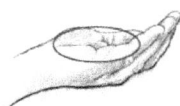

1 ounce
1 serving of
- snack food
- cheese (1 slice)

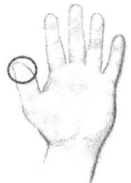

1 tablespoon
1 serving of
- salad dressing
- cream cheese

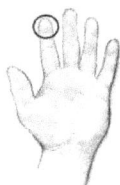

1 teaspoon
1 serving of
- margarine or butter
- oil
- mayonnaise

When You're Sick

Take care of yourself when you're sick. Being sick can make your blood glucose go too high. Tips on what to do include the following:

- Check your blood glucose level every 4 hours. Write down the results.

- Keep taking your diabetes medicines. You need them even if you can't keep food down.

- Drink at least one cup (8 ounces) of water or other calorie-free, caffeine-free liquid every hour while you're awake.

- If you can't eat your usual food, try drinking juice or eating crackers, popsicles, or soup.

- If you can't eat at all, drink clear liquids such as ginger ale. Eat or drink something with sugar in it if you have trouble keeping food down, because you still need calories. If you can't eat enough, you increase your risk of low blood glucose, also called hypoglycemia.

- In people with type 1 diabetes, when blood glucose is high, the body produces ketones. Ketones can make you sick. Test your urine or blood for ketones if
  - your blood glucose is above 240
  - you can't keep food or liquids down

- Call your health care provider right away if
  - your blood glucose has been above 240 for longer than a day
  - you have ketones
  - you feel sleepier than usual
  - you have trouble breathing
  - you can't think clearly
  - you throw up more than once
  - you've had diarrhea for more than 6 hours

Where can I get more information?

Diabetes Teachers (nurses, dietitians, pharmacists, and other health professionals)

To find a diabetes teacher near you, call the American Association of Diabetes Educators toll-free at 1–800–TEAMUP4 (832–6874) or see *www.diabeteseducator.org* and click on "Find an Educator."

Recognized Diabetes Education Programs (teaching programs approved by the American Diabetes Association)

To find a program near you, call the American Diabetes Association toll-free at 1–800–DIABETES (342–2383) or see *www.diabetes.org/education/edustate2.asp* on the Internet.

Dietitians

To find a dietitian near you, call the American Dietetic Association's National Center for Nutrition and Dietetics toll-free at 1–800–877–1600 or see *www.eatright.org* and click on "Find a Nutrition Professional."

National Diabetes Information Clearinghouse

1 Information Way
Bethesda, MD 20892–3560
Phone: 1–800–860–8747
Fax: 703–738–4929
Email: ndic@info.niddk.nih.gov
Internet: www.diabetes.niddk.nih.gov

The National Diabetes Information Clearinghouse (NDIC) is a service of the National Institute of Diabetes and Digestive and Kidney Diseases (NIDDK). The NIDDK is part of the National Institutes of Health under the U.S. Department of Health and Human Services. Established in 1978, the Clearinghouse provides information about diabetes to people with diabetes and to their families, health care professionals, and the public. The NDIC answers inquiries, develops and distributes publications, and works closely with professional and patient organizations and Government agencies to coordinate resources about diabetes.

Publications produced by the Clearinghouse are carefully reviewed by both NIDDK scientists and outside experts. This booklet was originally reviewed by Marion J. Franz, M.S., R.D., L.D., C.D.E., Minneapolis, and Carolyn Leontos, M.S., R.D., C.D.E., University of Nevada.

This publication may contain information about medications used to treat a health condition. When this publication was prepared, the NIDDK included the most current information available. Occasionally, new information about medication is released. For updates or for questions about any medications, please contact the U.S. Food and Drug Adminstration at 1–888–INFO–FDA (463–6332), a toll-free call, or visit their website at *www.fda.gov.* Consult your doctor for more information.

www.ingramcontent.com/pod-product-compliance
Lightning Source LLC
Chambersburg PA
CBHW081356170526
45166CB00010B/3111